I0484264

Everything You Need To Know About LASIK

A Patient's Guide To Refractive Surgery

Richard N. Gordon, M.D.
Medical Director
Palisades Laser Eye Center
Pomona, New York
Clinical Associate Adjunct Professor
The New York Eye & Ear Infirmary of Mount Sinai
New York, New York

Copyright 2014, Richard N. Gordon, M.D.

Title Disclaimer: *"Well, maybe not everything..."*

Although the title is of this book is true for most patients, every rule has exceptions, all medical procedures are complex, and each patient is unique. Each reader may have their own opinion about what they need to know. Readers should take the title with a grain of salt and use this book as described in the Introduction.

Table of Contents

Introduction

Over the course of my career, I have performed thousands of laser refractive procedures. I have also been one of those who benefited from the surgery, a patient on the other side of the laser, so to speak. My patients have been moms and grand moms, doctors and lawyers, truck drivers and hairdressers, in short someone just like you. For every single patient I see in consultation, much of the time spent involves me educating them about what refractive surgery is as well as its risks and benefits. I am sometimes surprised how many patients try to make the decision whether or not to choose such a wonderful and life-changing event without making the effort to become more familiar with the basic information they should know first.

Just type "LASIK" into any internet search engine, and you will be inundated with links to sources about the procedure. Although these reports may be great at sparking interest in prospective patients, or possibly dissuading them with ranting descriptions of perceived complications, they are often not accurate and certainly not to be trusted as a definitive source. Every patient is different, and thus their potential outcome can be different as well. When I hear the misinformation prospective patients have gleaned from others, it reminds me of the children's game, Telephone, where the words get slightly distorted as they are passed on from person to person. The reality is that even the best possible results are individualized, and you should not base your expectations only on the results of others.

This book is written to give you the same information I try to give my patients during a consultation. It should not be considered a definitive source but more of a guide to help you understand the process of refractive surgery. At the very least, you'll want to note down questions for discussion and any points of misunderstanding. Before you can judge whether or not the surgery is for you, understanding how the eye works to focus light, called "optics," is very helpful. The first chapter teaches you just the basic optics required to know precisely what "nearsightedness", "farsightedness", and "astigmatism", are, for example. Chapter 2 will describe how laser refractive surgery treats these conditions and what its limitations are. Chapter 3 will discuss the possible risks in the categories of side effects, minor complications, and major complications. Chapter 4 will tell you what to expect before, during, and after your procedure. Chapter 5 helps clarify some of the options you have in *how* the procedure is performed. By the end, you will have enough working knowledge of this kind of surgery to make a good—and well-informed—choice. Of course, as with any surgical procedure, you should make sure all of your questions are answered, then all you need is a thorough exam, and you should be ready to go!

Chapter 1: Basic Optics

To understand how refractive surgery can help improve your vision, first you need to know how it changes the way your eye focuses light. To begin, we'll look at how the various parts of the eye involved function to accomplish that task. This is one part of a broader, subject called "Optics."

No, you don't need a full course in Optics, and my intention here is to give you just what you need to know in an easy-to-comprehend way. Familiarizing yourself with a few basic concepts will help you understand what a refractive surgeon does and why, and better educate you about your own choices and what to expect. The great thing is that, while you don't need to put in the years of study like I did, understanding light, vision, and how the eye works is actually pretty fascinating. (If you want to study further after you read this, I would recommend the textbook *Optics for Clinicians* by Melvin Rubin[1].)

Optics describes how light is focused. Light is somewhat of an enigma in science; even physicists have trouble describing it. For instance, depending on the circumstances, it can behave as a particle or a wave. For our purposes, we only need to think of it as being a kind of energy made up of "rays." Imagine the light coming from any source, like the sun or a light bulb, as countless beams of energy shooting in all directions [2] (Figure 1). These beams, or rays, travel in straight lines away from their source, so they naturally spread apart, or diverge, from each other the farther away they are from the source. This is called "divergence."

[1]Rubin, M. (1974). *Optics for Clinicians*. Gainesville, Fla.: Triad Scientific Publishers.
[2]Rubin, M. (1974). *Optics for Clinicians*. Gainesville, Fla.: Triad Scientific Publishers, page 3.

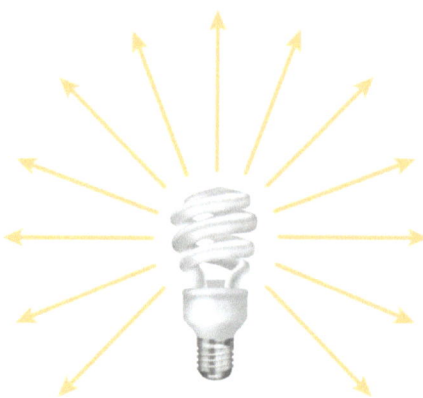

Figure 1: Light rays diverge from a light source because they travel in straight lines.

When light rays from a source such as the sun or a light bulb hit an object, the light rays bounce, or "reflect" off the object. These reflected light rays act the same way as light from its original source, namely, diverging from each other in all directions (Figure 2).

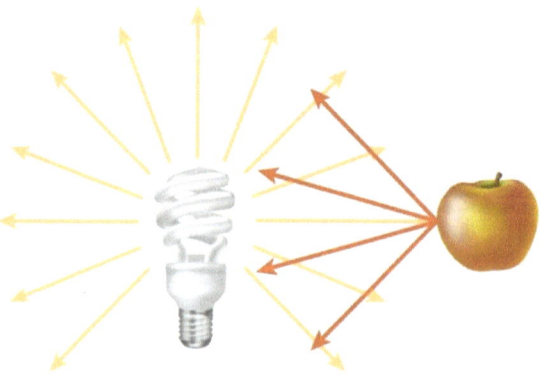

Figure 2: Light rays that reflect off an object also diverge from the point of reflection.

To see this object at all, your eye must capture these reflected light rays. But to see the object *clearly*, your eye must manipulate the light rays, bending them back down to a single point. A basic property of light is that when it passes through a transparent flat surface, like the glass in a window pane, the rays go through straight. But when the surface is curved, the light rays are redirected (Figure 3).

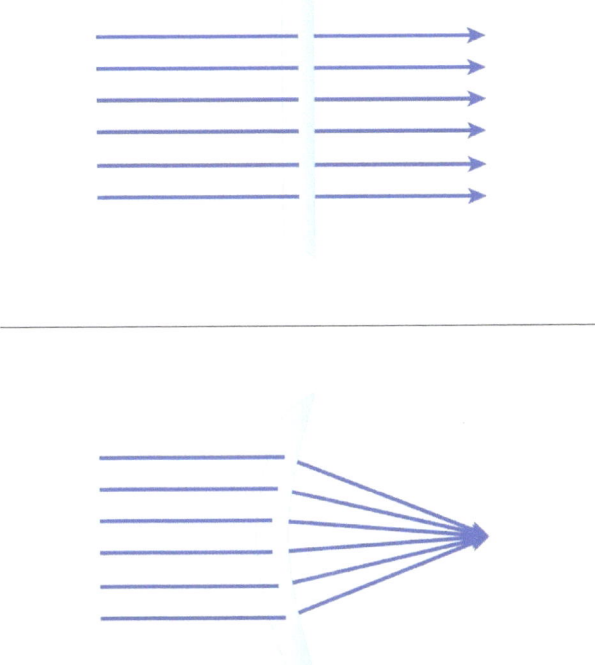

Figure 3: Light rays passing through a flat surface are not changed, but light rays traveling through a curved surface are bent.

Bending light rays causes them to come back together, or "converge" to a point; we define this as the process of "focusing," and for this discussion, we will call the point the light rays converge on as the "focal point" (Figure 4).

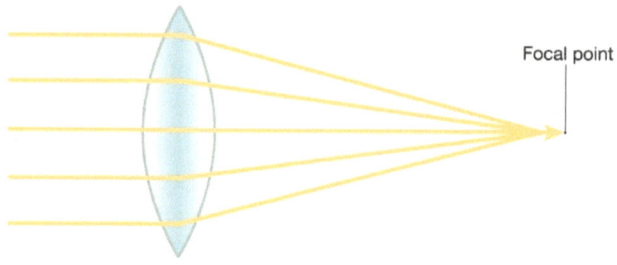

Figure 4: A curved surface bends incoming light rays so that they converge at a focal point.

So how does your eye bend the reflected light rays to the focal point? Well, your eye has two special parts, the cornea and the lens, that bend the light (Figure 5).

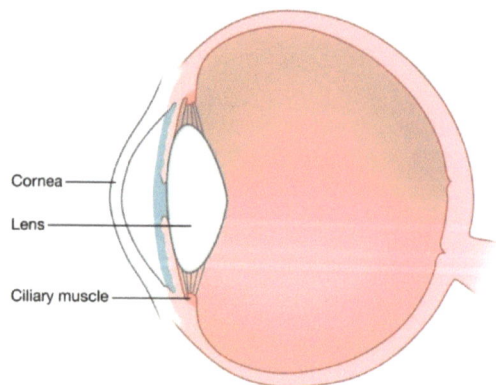

Figure 5: The cornea and lens focus incoming light in the eye.

The more curved a surface, the more it bends light. The curve of the cornea, its shape, is fixed; it does not change. In other words, the cornea focuses light to the same degree all the time. The lens of the eye, however, is attached to the ciliary muscle and that muscle can make the lens more or less curved. When the muscle is relaxed, the lens is somewhat flat and not too powerful. When the muscle contracts, the lens of your eye becomes more curved and thus has additional focusing power. (Figure 6).

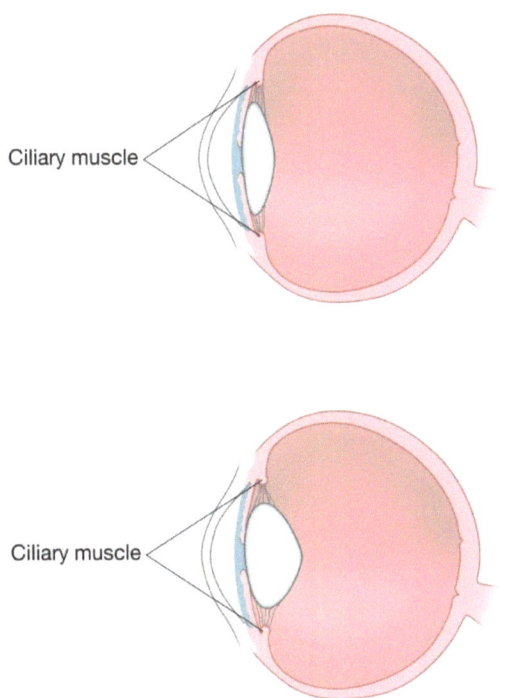

Figure 6: When the ciliary muscle contracts, the lens becomes more curved and is able to focus light even more.

We need to consider one last thing before putting this all together and figuring out how the eye works. This is the distance between our eye and the object we're looking at. Objects up close, say within arm's length, reflect more light rays to the eye than an object far away (Figure 7). As you can see from the diagram, many of those light rays have a very divergent angle to the eye. But when an object is far enough away, say 20 feet, only the light rays that are *not* diverging reach the eye. Since these light rays are traveling straight on, they need to be bent the least to reach the focal point (Figure 7).

If this is confusing for you, for simplicity, just remember that a distant object reflects light rays that reach the eye straight on, requiring less focusing effort *because* they are straight. In contrast, a near object reflects light rays that are directed away from the eye and have to be bent more to focus them. Closer objects thus require more focusing power.

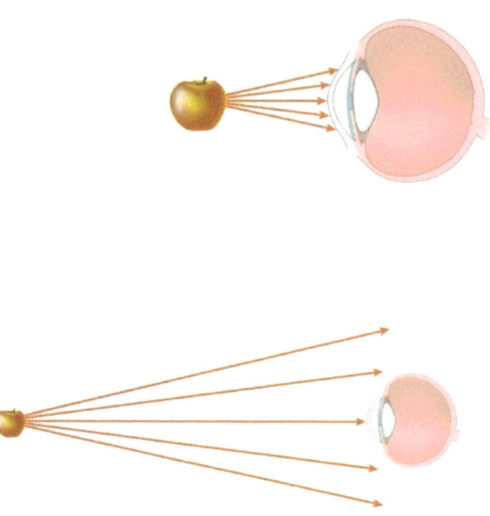

Figure 7: For a near object, most reflected light rays, including the diverging ones, reach the eye. For a distant object, only the reflected light rays that travel straight to the eye reach it, the diverging ones have spread apart so much they miss the eye. *More focusing is needed for a near object than a distant one.*

Okay, so now let's put it all together. Let's look at how the normal eye works and then examine the problems with eyes that don't see well at all distances.

Emmetropia

An eye is in *emmetropia* when it does not need glasses or contact lenses to see a **distant** object clearly. Remember, light rays reflected from the distant object hit the eye straight on, with no divergence. The cornea and lens bend those light rays to the focal point. The retina is the tissue in the in the back of your eye that processes the light and sends the signal to the brain. As long as the focal point is on the retina, a clear image is sent to the brain and the image is perceived as clear (Figure 8). When an emmetropic eye tries to see something in the distance, the ciliary muscle in the eye is relaxed. If the object is moved closer to the eye, more divergent light rays reach the eye, and more focusing power is needed. That is where the lens of the eye comes in. When the object is brought up close, your brain senses that it is not in focus. The brain then stimulates the muscle in the eye to contract, the lens becomes more curved, and the right amount of additional focus is added, moving the focal point to the retina for a "clear" picture, so to speak. This is called *accommodation* (Figure 8).

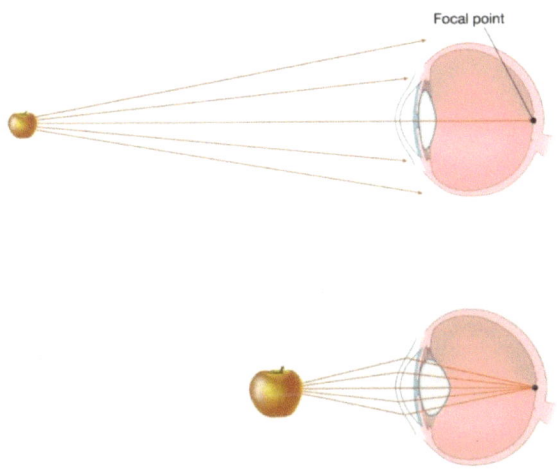

Figure 8: Emmetropia. The focal point for distant objects with the ciliary muscle relaxed is on the retina. For near objects, the

muscle contracts, and the lens becomes more curved and "accommodates" to focus the divergent light rays that now reach the eye.

What if your eye does not see well? Isn't that what this book is about? Absolutely! When an eye has trouble seeing but this trouble can be corrected with glasses, contact lenses, or surgery, it has what is called a *refractive error*. Here are the four major types of refractive errors.

Nearsightedness

When someone is nearsighted, or *myopic*, their eye is "longer" so that the focal point of light rays for a distant object is in front of the retina (Figure 8). ("Longer" just means that the distance between the cornea/lens and the retina is greater than normal.) The light rays then continue through the focal point and hit the retina but spread out, causing a blurry image. If you move the distant object closer to the eye, the focal point moves back as well until eventually it hits the retina and the object is clear (Figure 9).

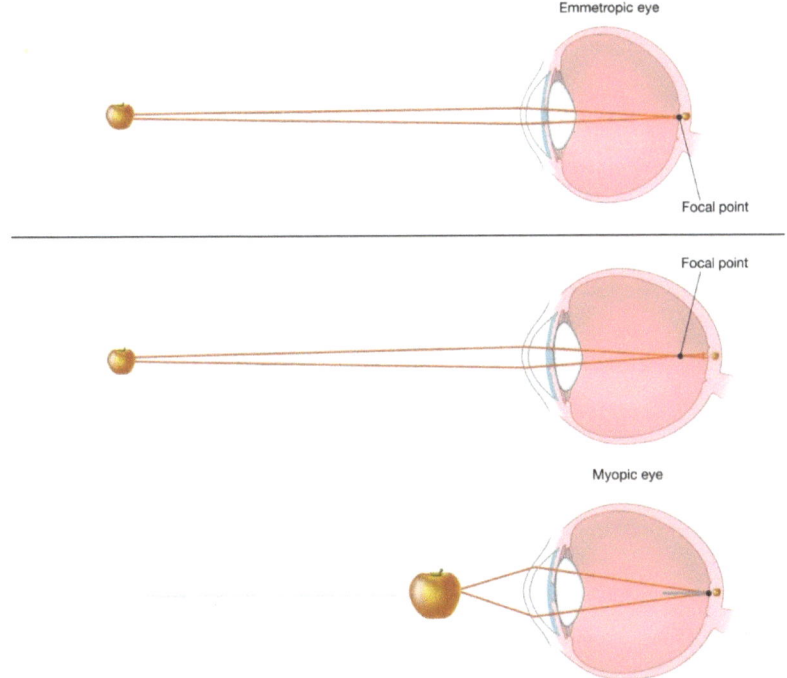

Figure 9: Emmetropic eye on top, myopic below. The myopic eye is longer so the focal point is in front of the retina. Light rays that reflect from a distant object pass through the focal point and reach the retina spread out so the image is fuzzy. If the object is moved closer to the eye, the focal point moves back until it hits the retina and the object appears clear and sharp.

If the object moves even closer to the eye after it comes into focus, the lens then kicks in to bring the object into focus. So a nearsighted person who is not wearing their glasses or contacts does not have to use their focusing muscle as much as an emmetropic person.

Farsightedness

When someone is farsighted, or *hyperopic*, their eye is shorter than an emmetropic eye, the opposite of nearsightedness. ("Shorter" here just means that the distance between the cornea/lens and the back of the eye is less than normal.) Since the eye is shorter, the focal point for a distant object is behind the retina (Figure 10). However, the eye has a way of adding extra focusing power to bring the focal point back onto the retina by flexing the muscle usually used for focusing on an object up close.

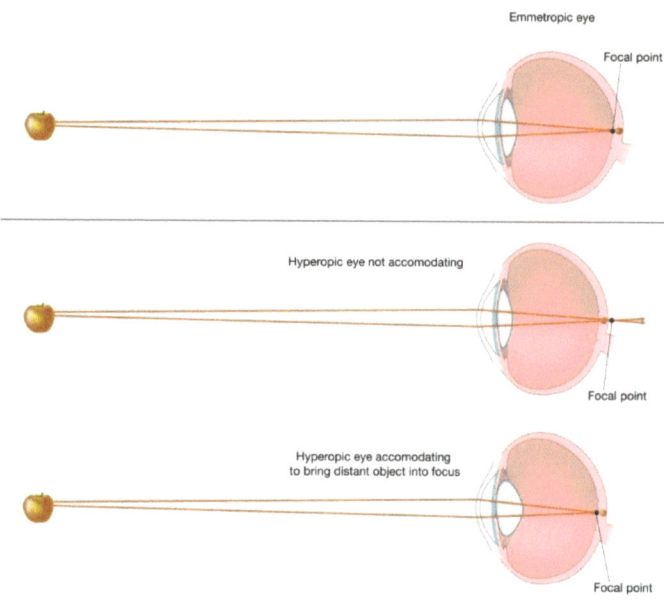

Figure 10: Emmetropic eye above, hyperopic below. The hyperopic eye is shorter, so the focal point for reflected light from a distant object falls behind the retina. Since the focal point is behind the retina, the object is blurry. The eye will accommodate to increase the lens power and bring the focal point onto the retina.

The problem is that each eye has a limit to its focusing power, and a farsighted person is using some of that power just to see a distant object. So a farsighted person may be able to see a distant object like an emmetropic person but will then have to work harder to see an up close object without extra help from glasses. If a person is farsighted enough, the eye will not have enough focusing power even to bring light rays from a distant object onto the retina, and it will be blurry. Thus, they might need glasses for distance as well as near vision. (Of course, for many people, bifocals are a common solution.)

Astigmatism

This is the one term most commonly misunderstood by my patients. Most people can figure out that a nearsighted person can see up close, and a farsighted person can see far away, but what does astigmatism mean? Let's use a definition of astigmatism simplified a bit so we can all understand how it affects the eye. **All you need to know is that an eye with astigmatism has an oval shaped cornea compared to a normal eye with a spherical cornea.** Remember, the amount of curvature of a surface dictates how much focusing power, or light bending ability, it has. When the curvature of the cornea is perfectly uniform like the surface of a basketball, wherever light hits it, the cornea will bend the light to the same degree (Figure 11). However, if the cornea has an oval shape more like a football, the shorter axis of the oval—the very roundest part of the ball around its center—has more curvature than the longer axis, towards the tips (Figure 11).

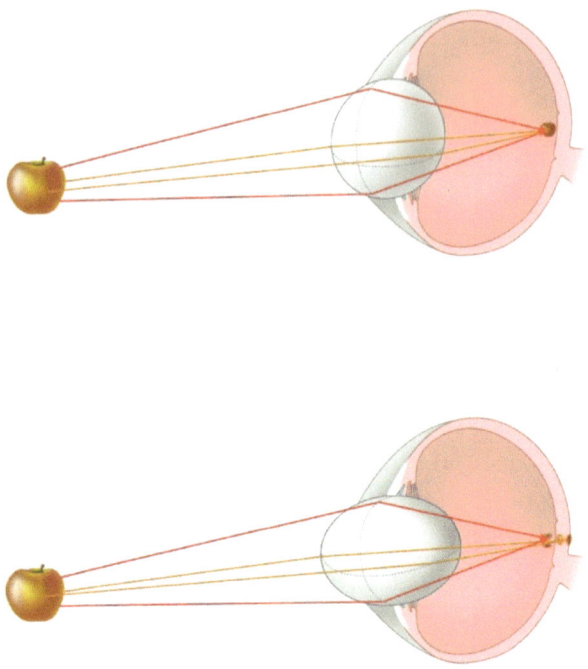

Figure 11: Spherical-shaped cornea on top, oval-shaped cornea on the bottom. For the spherical cornea, light is focused the same amount wherever it hits the cornea because the curvature is the same all over. For the oval cornea, the longer part is less curved and bends light less than the shorter part. There is no single focal point and so the image appears blurry.

This unequal curvature causes the focal point of the eye to be spread out instead of being a sharp point because the rays are not all being focused on the same single spot. Ophthalmologists say an eye with a round cornea is spherical, and an eye with an oval cornea is *astigmatic*. Note, too, that people can have a combination of nearsightedness with astigmatism, or farsightedness with astigmatism (Figure 12).

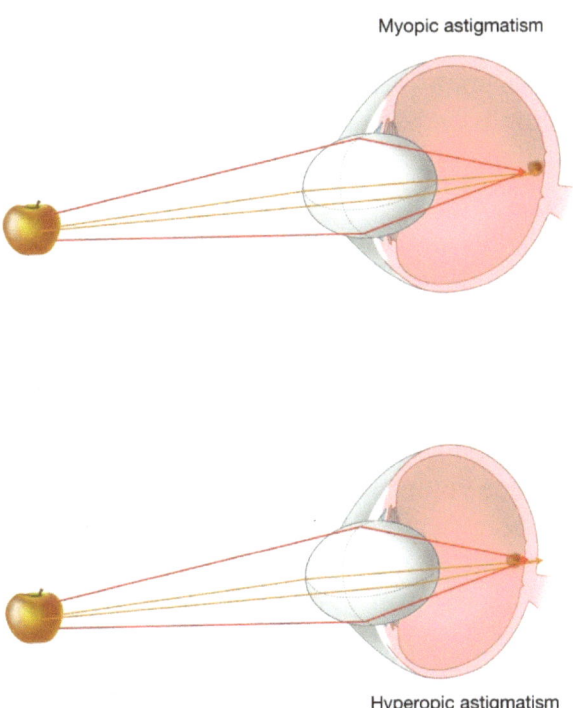

Figure 12: An eye with myopic astigmatism is longer and has an oval-shaped cornea. An eye with hyperopic astigmatism is shorter and has oval-shaped cornea.

Presbyopia

This is the last cause of blurry vision we need to consider, and it is also frequently misunderstood. Though many people mistakenly confuse presbyopia with all three of the problems we discussed above, it is completely different from them. It has nothing to do with how long the eye is or how curved the cornea is. Presbyopia occurs in everyone. It happens as we get older. With time, the lens of the eye starts to become stiffer and does not flex as much. So it cannot respond as well to the focusing action of the ciliary muscle. Remember, the lens needs to become more curved to add focusing power to the eye for near objects. When presbyopia occurs, people typically have more difficulty seeing an up close object than when they were younger. Believe it or not, people start losing their focusing power in their late teens, but they usually don't notice it until their mid-forties. It continues, unrelentingly, until the lens barely responds to the muscle at all, usually when people reach their mid-seventies.

Remember, a myopic eye does not have to start accommodating with additional focusing power until the object moves closer. Conversely, a hyperopic person will notice presbyopia sooner than an emmetropic person because the former are usually accommodating for distance and near vision.

These are the basic concepts behind the various kinds of blurry vision. Once you understand them and know which apply to you, together we can figure out the best treatment for you. We'll look at all the various options in the next chapter. If you are still not sure about the different types of refractive error, try re-reading the chapter. You might want to refer back to it as needed as you read the next chapters.

Chapter 2: The Benefits of Refractive Surgery

Now that we have a basic understanding of how a normal eye sees a distant and a near object, and the reasons for refractive errors leading to poor or blurry vision, let's look at how we treat these conditions.

We have three ways to treat refractive errors:
1. Eyeglasses with Corrective Lenses
2. Contact Lenses
3. Refractive Surgery

That's it! These are the three tools we have for treatment. Though most people with refractive errors are familiar with glasses and contacts, they don't really know how each works. Refractive surgery is even more of a mystery.

Before we get into the actual treatments, we need to learn a little more about *refractive surgery*, which is any surgery that corrects a refractive error in the eye.   Several types of refractive surgery exist. Refractive surgery performed on the cornea is the most popular and widely performed type of refractive surgery. It makes sense to operate on the cornea as it is right on the surface of the eye and so is easy to access.

The two major types of refractive surgery on the cornea are LASIK, Laser-Assisted In-Situ Keratomileusis, and PRK, or Photo Refractive Keratectomy. You don't necessarily need to remember what each stands for, so let's just call them LASIK and PRK. The major difference is that, in LASIK, a thin flap is made on the cornea, and a laser is used to change the shape of the cornea under the flap. In PRK, no flap is made; the laser works right on the surface to change the shape of the cornea, which then heals by itself (Figure 13)

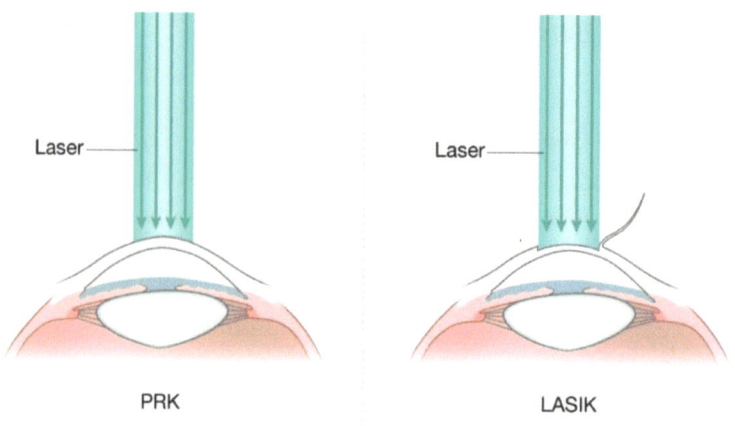

Figure 13: For PRK, laser energy is applied to the surface of the cornea to change its curvature. In LASIK, a thin flap of cornea is first made and the same laser energy is applied to inner layers underneath.

We will get into more details about LASIK and PRK later. For now, just know that they both do the same thing; they change the curvature of the cornea.

The other major type of refractive surgery ignores the cornea and works by replacing the lens or adding additional lens implants inside the eye (Figure 14).

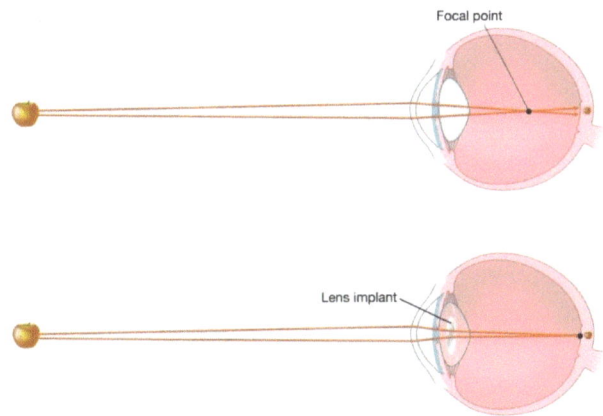

Figure 14: Lens-based refractive surgery changes the focusing power of the eye by placing lens implants into the eye.

It is more invasive because the surgeon has to gain access to the inside of the eye. We call these procedures *intraocular* precisely because they take place inside the eye. We will talk mostly about corneal refractive surgery, but we will also touch on lens-based, intraocular surgery as well.

All right, so how do we correct refractive errors? First, let's discuss how to treat the three types of refractive errors that affect the eye's focusing of a *distant* object; myopia, hyperopia, and astigmatism.

Myopia

Remember from the last chapter that, when someone is myopic, or nearsighted, the focal point for the eye for a distant object is in front of the retina because the eye is long. If we decrease the focusing power of the eye, we can move the focal point onto the retina. Glasses and contact lenses do this by redirecting the light rays before they reach the eye (Figure 15).

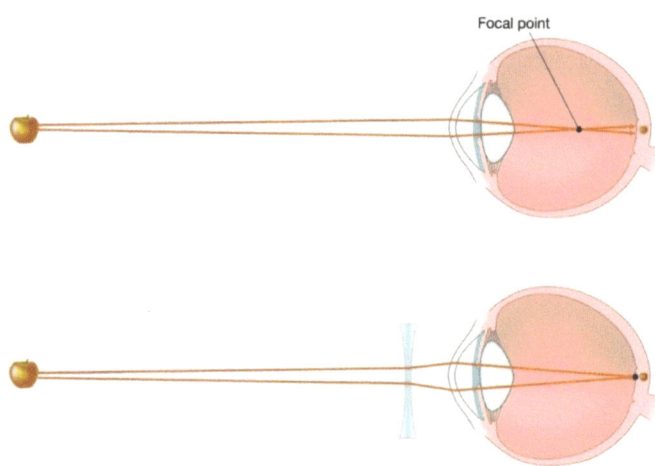

Figure 15: An eyeglass or contact lens placed in front, or on the surface of, the eye redirects incoming light rays so the focal point is moved back, onto the retina and the image is clear.

The purpose of corneal refractive surgery is to change the shape of the cornea. For myopia, it will flatten the cornea to decrease the focusing power of the eye, thus decreasing the converging power of the cornea and moving the focal point onto the retina (Figure 16).

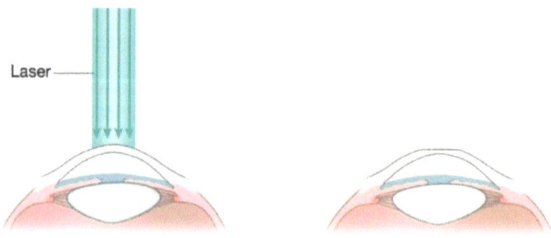

Figure 16: For corneal laser surgery to correct myopia, the laser flattens the central part of the cornea.

Hyperopia

Let's also recall from the last chapter that hyperopia, or farsightedness, causes a distant object to be focused behind the retina because the eye is short. To correct this, glasses and contact lenses redirect the incoming light rays and add convergence to them to move the focal point onto the retina. Corneal refractive surgery for farsightedness increases the curvature of the cornea—make it steeper—adding converging power to the cornea to move the focal point onto the retina (Figure 17).

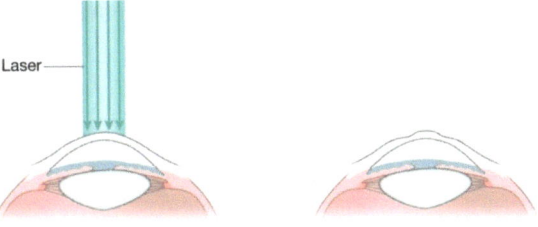

Figure 17: Laser surgery on the cornea to correct hyperopia steepens the central cornea making it more curved and thus more powerful.

Astigmatism

With astigmatism, remember, the cornea is oval-shaped, causing the focal point to be spread out. Glasses and contact lenses correct astigmatism by using an oval lens oriented to neutralize the astigmatism (Figure 18).

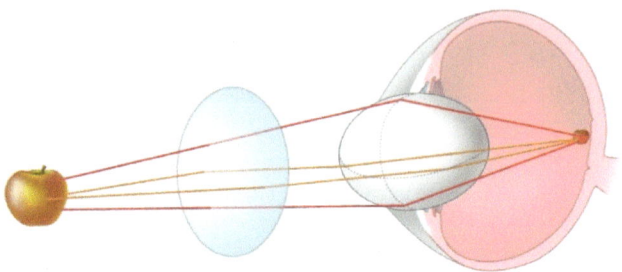

Figure 18: An oval-shaped lens correcting astigmatism.

Corneal refractive surgery corrects astigmatism by making the central part of the cornea more spherical (Figure 19).

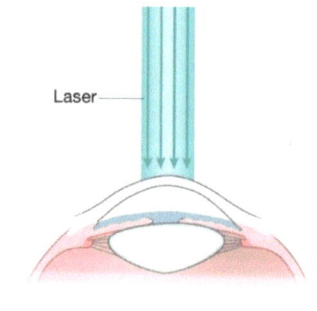

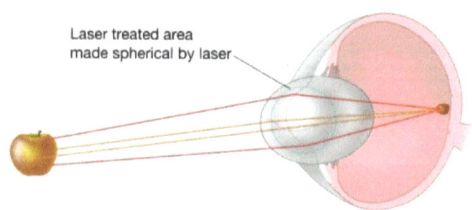

Figure 19: Top, laser making the central cornea more spherical and, bottom, correcting astigmatism.

The primary benefit of corneal refractive surgery in the procedures above is to provide equivalent quality of vision for a *distant* object as you get with glasses or contact lenses. The key to understanding this benefit is that it applies to *distant objects only.* A reasonable expectation of refractive surgery is to see objects as well in the distance as you see them wearing your glasses and contact lenses.

Now, here's something interesting. A good way to simulate the effect of corneal refractive surgery is simply to put on your distance glasses! Now that you understand that light rays coming from a distant object needs to be focused differently than light rays coming from a near object, this point should be apparent. Don't try to figure out what the effect of refractive surgery will be on near vision just by taking your distance glasses off. For example, if you take off your distance glasses to see something up close, do not use this as a guide for what corneal refractive surgery can do for you. You'll understand more about why this is when we describe how to correct near vision difficulty, or presbyopia, below.

Presbyopia

Remember, presbyopia occurs when the lens inside the eye becomes stiffer and can't change its shape to sufficient degree to add convergence, or extra focusing power, to the eye. When presbyopia occurs, people compensate for it in different ways. If they see distant objects well , they usually add focusing power to the eye with near vision glasses. If they are hyperopic, farsighted, they will probably need to start using near vision glasses sooner than someone who is emmetropic, or of normal vision. A myopic, nearsighted, person can see something up close without using the focusing power of the lens if they do not wear their distant correction, so they can sometimes take their distant glasses off to see up close, in reading a book, for example.

Other ways to correct presbyopia blend distant and near corrections. Bifocal glasses have distant correction on the top of the lenses and more focusing power on the bottom. Bifocal contact lenses have two focusing powers built into them as well. Other contact lens wearers wear so-called monovision lenses where one eye is corrected for distance vision and the other is corrected for near vision. All of these blended corrective measures can compromise the overall quality of vision somewhat. For example, with monovision, because both eyes are not fully focused on the object at the same time, depth perception is diminished. Yet the advantage of course, is that you don't have to have multiple pairs of glasses, or different lenses, when looking at an object up close.

I always find that my happiest patients are those who have a clear understanding of what to expect from refractive surgery. And so I usually spend a lot of time not only discussing what refractive surgery *can* do but what it *cannot* do as well. *The simple truth is that corneal refractive surgery does not do a great job of correcting presbyopia.*

As we've learned, corneal refractive surgery can correct refractive errors for distant light rays very, very well. But remember that the cornea cannot change its curvature; it will bend incoming light rays the same no matter their angle of approach. Since light rays for a near object reach the eye differently than light rays for a distant object, how can a person expect the cornea to focus those rays as well?

You have probably figured out by now that, quite simply, the cornea cannot do it all. Sometimes this fact comes as quite a surprise to my patients during a consultation. Maybe they have seen some fantastic advertising promising them that they will "throw their glasses away." Many of the readers of this book may have seen such misleading claims. While patients pretty much can be rid of *distance* glasses or contacts after corneal refractive surgery, they will still need *something* for near vision, when they reach the age when presbyopia sets in.

So are myopic, hyperopic, and/or astigmatic patients who are also presbyopic still candidates for corneal refractive surgery? Absolutely. They just have to understand that they will need something for near vision after refractive surgery. The easiest option is just to wear near vision spectacles, and in most cases inexpensive over the counter glasses work well. My own story illustrates this and might be of interest to you. I had LASIK surgery over fifteen years ago for myopia and had no need for glasses of any kind—until recently. When I reached my mid-forties and presbyopia started creeping in, I had to adjust. Now I wear over-the-counter magnifiers when I need them. I certainly don't consider the original surgery a failure or that the surgery is "wearing off." I understand that what is going on inside my eye is quite simply the natural effects of aging and something that corneal refractive surgery cannot treat.

The other option for presbyopic patients who choose corneal refractive surgery is monovision. Just as with contact lenses, we can aim for monovision after refractive surgery where one eye is treated so as to improve focus on distant objects and one treated to better focus on near objects. If you are considering this, you should understand that you may be compromising both distance and near vision somewhat. As we learned earlier, depth perception is decreased with monovision, and your brain needs to adjust to one eye being less clear than the other. For patients who have not tried monovision before, I will always help them simulate what the result will be with a contact lens trial before proceeding with surgery to see if they can tolerate it.

Patients who choose monovision also need to understand that even if they do well initially, as the presbyopia gets worse with time (as it does in all of us), they may become symptomatic again and need more help with up close vision. I usually discourage additional laser surgery for these cases because the presbyopia will continue, and higher levels of monovision are usually not well tolerated because most people cannot get used to the greater difference between the two eyes required at that point.

A new technology is emerging to address this shortcoming by placing a near-vision implant beneath a LASIK flap. It is not yet

FDA approved in the United States, however, and most American surgeons have minimal experience with it. It too requires optical compromises but may be better tolerated than monovision. The jury is still out on these corneal implants.

The final surgical option for presbyopic candidates is lens-based, intraocular surgery. Intraocular, remember, means surgery actually on the inside, rather than the surface parts, of the eye. Several intraocular lens implants have the ability to focus on both near and distant objects to some degree. Cataract surgery is intraocular and involves removing the lens of the eye and replacing it with an implant, or artificial lens, and I always discuss this option with my patients when I discover a cataract during a consultation. As I wrote earlier, intraocular surgery is more invasive with a whole different set of benefits and risks, a discussion beyond the scope of this book. Some, very few, patients do insist that, if there is an option such that, after surgery, they will not need any kind of glasses or contact lenses, that is the choice for them. For these individuals, some type of intraocular lens, possibly combined with corneal refractive surgery, will be necessary.

The last concept that prospective refractive surgery patients need to understand is that the lens inside your eye changes with time. We already discussed how the lens becomes less flexible with normal aging, causing presbyopia. The next change in the lens occurs when the proteins in the lens change. When we are born, the lens is clear, almost like glass. As we grow older, the proteins change, the lens becoming yellow to brown in color with the result that light does not pass through it as well. Once the lens starts to change, we call it a cataractous lens or a *cataract* for short. Cataracts are not a film growing inside the eye as some patients think but rather a change in the lens itself. Cataracts happen to all of us to some degree if we live long enough.

Not all cataracts are dense enough to affect vision. However, when they do affect vision in a patient who has had previous corneal refractive surgery, I've often heard him or her tell me that they have the feeling the original surgery is "wearing off." Almost every week I will get a call from a patient who had corneal refractive surgery in the past who has either a cataract or presbyopia and who wants some additional corneal refractive surgery done to compensate for it as a "touch up." Except under very rare cases, the cornea does not change much with time, even after LASIK or PRK. The change people experience with time after such procedures is almost always due to the inevitable change in the lens of the eye. I resist performing additional surgery on the cornea due to progressive changes in the lens; this is sort of like a dog chasing his tail because the lens will continue to change with time.

Patients who develop changes in the lens of their eye but are not ready for intraocular surgery usually do quite well with glasses or more rarely contact lenses for the few times in the day that additional focusing is needed. I always tell corneal refractive surgery patients that they should *not* consider the use of glasses from time to time or to watch their favorite sports team as a failure of the original surgery. In fact, they should expect it at some point. Most patients who experience these changes usually are concerned that their vision will revert completely back to their pre-LASIK or PRK levels and usually just need reassurance that this is not the case. These slight changes in vision are normal and happen to all of us over time.

So, to sum this all up, refractive surgery is most commonly performed on the cornea and does a great job of correcting distant vision problems. Normal changes to the lens inside the eye will occur with time and should be expected. Several options exist for dealing with these changes, including other surgeries, but none of them are perfect. The bottom line is that refractive surgery patients should adjust their expectations. If they believe that they will never need glasses or contact lenses again for any reason for the rest of their lives, this is simply not realistic and will only lead to later disappointment.

Chapter 3: Risks of Refractive Surgery

By this point, I hope you have a basic understanding of how the eye works, how refractive surgery can correct refractive errors, and normal changes that can occur after corneal refractive surgery. Now let's consider what may happen if the unexpected occurs during or after surgery.

No one likes to consider risks, but the simple truth is that risk is a factor in all medical interventions, from the tests performed during a routine examination, to the prescription and use of even common medications, to surgical procedures. In fact, most activities in life have risk, like driving in a car, walking down stairs, skiing, or flying in an airplane. People don't usually think about it, but they risk their life just driving to my office for a consultation! Risk is a fact of life. However, just because an activity has risks associated with it does not necessarily mean it is inherently or highly *risky.*

Still, as a candidate for this surgery, you need to have a basic acceptance that complications can occur in any medical procedure. Corneal refractive surgery is no exception. In my opinion, the magnitude of complications—the seriousness of what can go wrong—in corneal refractive surgery is less than most eye surgeries, especially intraocular surgeries. Because corneal refractive surgery involves only the outside of the eye, it avoids contact with the sensitive structures inside the eye that cannot always be repaired.

In the following explanations, I will avoid quoting statistics and incidence rates as much as possible. Why? Incidence rates— how often something untoward happens—can vary widely depending on the study or report cited while complication rates usually decrease with time as doctors learn new ways to avoid them. Instead, I will try to use more general terms in describing the likelihood of a given complication. Also, considering every conceivable complication is beyond the scope of this book; the subject matter is too complicated and confusing. Instead, I will attempt to categorize the risks into logical divisions that cover the important issues. Therefore, you should not consider this book an all-inclusive, exhaustively-detailed source like a medical textbook but rather a useful guide.

Three basic types of complications can occur:

1. Side Effects
2. Minor Problems
3. Major Problems

Side Effects

A side effect is something, generally expected, that occurs as a result of a normal procedure. All ways of correcting refractive errors have limitations. Glasses use plastic lenses that can have aberrations or scratches in them that degrade an image and make it blurry. They can cause magnification problems or even just maddeningly slide down your nose! Contact lenses can cause dryness, irritation, and allergies, and they can move around on the cornea which causes an image to become degraded as well.

In my opinion, the side effects related to corneal refractive surgery are less bothersome than the degradations associated with glasses and contacts. I wore glasses and contacts before I had LASIK surgery, and the vast majority of my patients agree with me that the side effects of the surgery are far more preferable than with glasses or contacts. Still, you need to know what the four basic types of side effects are and why they can occur.

The first is dryness. No one knows precisely why people experience dry eye after refractive surgery. The prevailing theory is that some of the nerves that stimulate normal tear production on the surface of the cornea may be damaged by the surgery. Most of the nerves grow back, but they can take a few months to reach maximum density during which time your eyes can be drier than normal. Some studies have suggested that normal tear production can be slightly decreased for years after corneal refractive surgery. In my experience, this dryness is most notable in the first few weeks or months after surgery, with tear production in most patients returning to normal after that. Most patients who complain of chronic dry eye *after* refractive surgery complained of dry eye *before* the surgery. This actually makes a lot of sense because many who seek out refractive surgery do so because they can't tolerate their contacts. Wearing the lenses, their eyes were too dry. Refractive surgery causes less dryness than contact lenses, and dry eye is treatable in a number of ways, from over-the-counter lubricating drops to prescription medications.

The next common side effect is night vision disturbances. Some patients complain about a glow or halo around images at night. This also is most pronounced immediately after surgery but fades as the swelling goes down. Again, we don't understand the precise cause of these disturbances. Probably, they have something to do with a combination of factors. One is the size of the area surgically treated as compared to the pupil. The pupil, like the aperture of a camera, can shrink or enlarge to let more or less light into the eye. In bright light, it becomes smaller, while at night it enlarges to let in as much light as possible. The laser correction is performed in a defined area on the cornea with a blending out to the periphery. When the pupil dilates widely at night, some light passes through the untreated area outside the correction and into the eye to cause these disturbances (Figure 20).

Day (normal pupil)

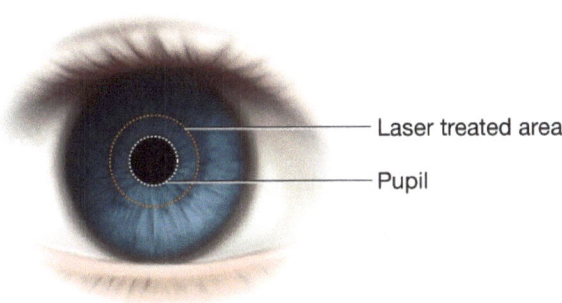

Laser treated area

Pupil

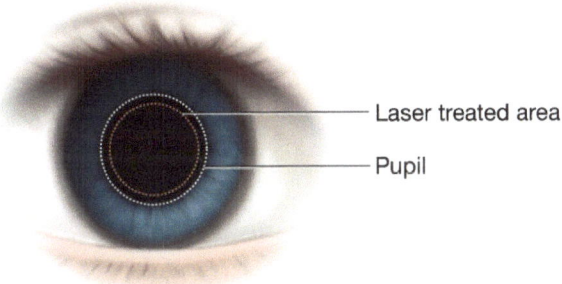

Laser treated area

Pupil

Night (dilated pupil)

Figure 20: Above: During the day, the pupil is small and light only passes through the treated central area of the cornea. Below: At night the pupil is dilated, so light enters the eye from the laser treated area (orange circle) and the untreated area beyond causing aberrations.

Night vision disturbances have been greatly diminished with improvements in laser technology. Such improvements include pupil tracking to more perfectly center the treatment, blending the treated area into the untreated area, treatments customized to individual eye shapes, sizes, and characteristics, and finally, iris registration. We will explore the meaning of all of these in the next chapter. Of course, contact lenses cause night vision disturbances, too, because the lens moves as you blink and so shifts the optical zone constantly. Interestingly, most contact lens wearers do not typically complain about night vision problems because they are usually less noticeable after corneal refractive surgery.

Another side effect is under- or overcorrection. Even though we can be very accurate in our preoperative measurements, some people respond to the same scope of laser treatment more than anticipated and some less so. The treatment's efficacy and final outcome can be affected by the cornea's water content, which is different for each person. The likelihood of a noticeable under- or over-correction also increases with the magnitude of that correction.

When an under-correction or over-correction is noticeable to the patient, I typically ask them to wait two to three months after the initial surgery before performing an additional surgery to address any residual refractive error. This is so that all healing has taken place and the touch-up will be as accurate as possible. As I mentioned in the previous chapter, enhancements should be reserved for patients who did not reach their target on the initial surgery. Patients who did reach the target but then notice a change years later most likely are experiencing something not surgery-related but due to some other change inside the eye that is not necessarily amenable to additional laser refractive surgery. These patients should discuss other options with their doctor.

Minor Problems

I classify a minor problem of corneal refractive surgery as something that will not significantly prevent good uncorrected vision after that problem is fully treated. A person who experiences a minor problem should expect to see about as well as if they did not have the problem after it is resolved. Some individuals just take longer to heal, and it may just be a question of more time after the surgery for them to get to that satisfactory vision. If you are in the middle of undergoing post-operative treatment, of course, the problem may not seem minor at all. This is especially true if you are comparing your result to a friend's in whose case no problems occurred. Still, most experienced refractive surgeons have seen the full gamut of minor problems and know how to treat them.

I mentioned earlier that two ways to perform corneal refractive surgery are PRK and LASIK. We will discuss later why patients may choose one over the other, but remember that in PRK, the laser is applied directly to the corneal surface which then heals. In LASIK, the surgeon first makes a flap on the corneal surface with the laser then applied underneath that flap. Each technique has its own minor problems.

In LASIK, such problems occur because of the flap—which must be both well-centered and large enough. If the surgeon does not feel that the flap is sufficient in size or quality to continue with surgery, he or she might replace it and abort the procedure. Sometimes, PRK then can be performed at that time instead, or later, after the flap has healed. Sometimes the flap is fine when it is created, but it heals with wrinkles, or cells grow underneath, or inflammation occurs. Many times, these problems go away with observation and eye drops. Rarely, the surgeon may have to re-lift the flap to treat them.

In PRK, minor problems can occur if the surface heals too aggressively and scar tissue—called "haze"—develops. Haze usually goes away with anti-inflammatory eye drops but occasionally needs to be removed manually or with the laser. Anti-scarring medications can be used at the time of surgery to help prevent haze.

Major Problems

At this point, many patients ask, "Okay, so what is the worst case scenario?" I classify these as major problems. A major problem after corneal refractive surgery can be treated to restore vision, but the treatment may involve more surgery. After treatment, the patient may need to wear contact lenses or eyeglasses again to achieve maximal vision. Though such surgery does come with risk, and a risk that each individual needs to recognize, the likelihood of permanent, un-correctable visual disability is extremely remote. Compare this to another common eye surgery, cataract surgery. This takes place inside the eye, and serious problems can occur which may not be correctable, such as damage to the retina or optic nerve. This does not occur typically with major corneal refractive surgery complications. These are relatively rare, and thankfully only two deserve consideration.

The first complication is infection. Both PRK and LASIK create an incision on the corneal surface which has to heal. Any surgical incision can become infected. Since PRK takes longer to heal than LASIK, the chance of an infection with PRK is probably slightly higher than with LASIK. If the infection is in the center of the cornea or particularly aggressive, it could leave a permanent scar that will affect vision.

Infections after refractive surgery are so rare that how often they occur is very difficult to measure accurately. In comparison, the likelihood of an infection from contact lenses is much higher. This makes sense because lens wearers are putting a foreign object on their eye for, at the very least, many hours every day. The risk of infection from surgery disappears after healing takes place. Contact lens wearers try to minimize the risk of infection by using disinfecting solutions for multiple-wear lenses or by using daily disposable lenses. A number of studies suggest that, even with these measures, any contact lens wearer likely assumes the risk of corneal infection to a much greater degree than that associated with corneal refractive surgery.

Every surgeon has their own regimen to prevent infections. I will usually ask patients to start prophylactic antibiotic eye drops a few days before the procedure and then for a week afterwards. I also perform the procedure with standard sterile surgical precautions. I ask my patients while they heal to stay out of high risk environments like hospitals or nursing homes where bacteria resistant to normal antibiotics can be found. I also suggest that friends or family who work in these higher-risk places wash their hands before coming into contact with a refractive surgery patient to avoid cross contamination. Contact lens wearers should discontinue use for a reasonable interval before surgery. I suggest a minimum of two weeks.

The other major complication is *ectasia*. To understand ectasia, patients need to remember that the laser used to reshape the cornea does so by removing corneal tissue to achieve the desired shape. This weakens the cornea slightly. Also, if a flap is made for LASIK, this flap weakens the cornea slightly as well. For the vast majority of patients who are normal, the cornea still has plenty of strength to maintain the desired shape, and this shape holds with minimal changes throughout the patient's life.

However, some people, estimated to be about one in two thousand, have a condition known as *keratoconus*, a genetic weakness of the cornea. The cornea of someone with keratoconus may not maintain the same shape throughout life, tending to bulge forward into a cone shape instead of the normal shape (Figure 21).

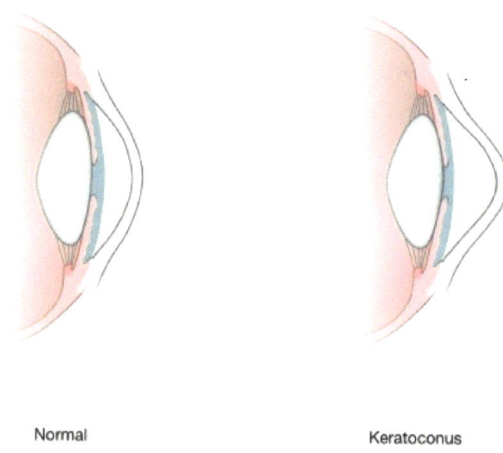

Normal   Keratoconus

Figure 21: Compared to a normal cornea, a cornea with keratoconus bulges forward into a cone shape.

The natural history of keratoconus is poorly understood. We don't know why some people progress to a more pronounced cone shape than others. Certainly, environmental factors may play a role. One environmental factor thought to contribute to keratoconus is eye rubbing. Forcefully rubbing an itchy eye increases the pressure inside the eye and strains the cornea. Over time, this may cause a cone to become more elevated. Eye rubbing can cause other eye problems as well, so I always caution my patients to avoid rubbing and to treat the cause of the itchiness, whether it is allergies, dry eye, or some other cause.

People with keratoconus already have a weaker cornea, and refractive surgery can weaken the cornea further. The surgery, therefore, could cause the cornea to become more cone shaped or to progress towards that at a more rapid rate. Since the cornea won't maintain the shape we are trying to achieve, these patients will not have ideal results. Obviously, we try hard to identify these patients during the pre-operative screening process. Some patients are easy to identify, but others have very subtle findings and may appear relatively normal.

The more experience we have with refractive surgery, the better we are at finding these difficult-to-identify patients. Patients with a family history of keratoconus in a direct relative like a sibling or parent are still at increased risk of developing the condition, even if their exam is completely normal. Patients with a very large correction, which thins the cornea more, may be at increased risk. Also, a person born with a very thin cornea may also have an increased risk of ectasia. Younger patients, those in their late teens and early twenties, may have a higher risk because the signs we are looking for may not yet be present. Having said all this, the degree to which these conditions increase the risk of ectasia is a hotly-debated topic among refractive surgeons, even to this day. Many well-respected refractive surgeons continue to present studies for and against performing surgery in patients with one or more of these conditions.

One condition that is widely accepted as the most important risk factor is the symmetry of the corneal shape. Refractive surgeons use very precise instruments to determine corneal shape and symmetry to help identify higher risk patients, and technology continues to improve. Still, many factors including dry eyes, chronic contact lens wear, and corneal scars make interpretation of these studies difficult. Even after these conditions are treated, interpretation still tends to be somewhat subjective. More sobering, even when everything is entirely normal and no risk factors are identified, some patients will still develop ectasia.

Since the flap in LASIK weakens the cornea slightly, performing surgery without a flap with PRK reduces the risk of ectasia. Again, every surgeon has his or her own criteria for which procedure to recommend to their patients, and prospective patients should discuss these options at length with their surgeon. Even though the post-operative recovery is longer with PRK, I recommend it to any of my patients who have increased risk factors but are still candidates for surgery. Although PRK does not eliminate the likelihood of ectasia, it does diminish it significantly. If everything is entirely normal, I usually recommend LASIK because the occurrence of ectasia is extremely rare and patients will recover sooner.

Even if ectasia does occur, today we have treatment options that maintain good vision without the need for major intraocular surgery. Years ago, the only treatments for ectasia were rigid contact lenses or a corneal transplant. We now have two procedures that strengthen the cornea and minimize the effects of ectasia. One is corneal ring segments, where the surgeon places semicircular rings in the cornea. The rings act as a brace and also flatten the central cone (Figure 22).

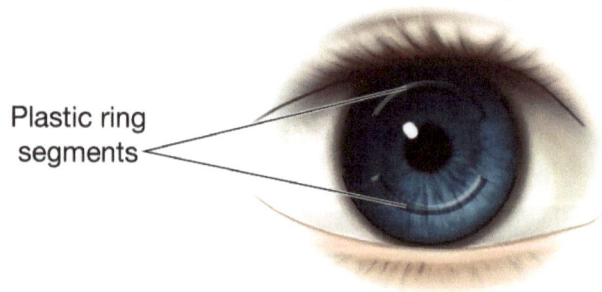

Plastic ring segments

Figure 22: Ring segments are placed in the cornea to treat ectasia/keratoconus.

The other exciting technology is collagen cross-linking, where the surgeon simply exposes the cornea to ultraviolet light. The light strengthens the cornea as much as 300%. Cross-linking can stop the ectasia progression and flatten the cone to reduce its severity. Many surgeons are combining these techniques and achieving results greater than either done singly. To further improve vision, surgeons in Europe and Asia have performed additional laser surgery to improve vision after the cross-linking has strengthened the cornea. The safety of this further treatment is still being evaluated in the United States but appears very promising.

While this chapter may be a little scary to read, its purpose is an important one. Remember, all surgery has some risk associated with it. Among the spectrum of medical procedures, however, corneal refractive surgery surely ranks among the safest. Even when problems occur, they almost always can be successfully managed and satisfactory vision maintained.

Chapter 4: Surgical Experience

Almost all patients are quite anxious about their refractive surgery. They can become preoccupied by questions like how long it takes, if it hurts, and how long they'll have to take medication after the procedure. The fear of the unknown can be quite profound, particularly when it involves something as important to us as our vision. After the experience is over, however, most patients realize that it was not nearly as terrible as their imaginations led them to believe. This chapter should help allay some of your concerns by describing what happens before, during, and after the surgery. All surgeons have their own unique regimen that works best for them, but these general guidelines should apply to the majority of procedures.

Before the Surgery: Preop

Thankfully, refractive surgery does not require much preparation on the part of the patient. Before the procedure, the patient should check with their general practitioner that they are healthy enough, but a formal clearance note or blood tests are not typically required. Routine medications that a patient may be taking typically do not need to be discontinued.

Some refractive surgeons will ask their patients to start using preoperative eye drops a few days before surgery. These drops may include an antibiotic to help reduce the risk of infection, an anti-inflammatory steroid drop to reduce swelling and scarring, and possibly an analgesic drop to reduce post-operative eye discomfort, or pain. Patients should also stop using their contact lenses as far ahead of the surgery as possible. Hard, gas-permeable contact lenses can alter the shape of the cornea and make the surgery less accurate, so the eye needs time free of these rigid contact lenses to return to its natural shape. This may take several weeks. Soft lenses do not typically alter the shape of the cornea, but they can cause dryness that can make preoperative examination of the cornea more difficult. Also, soft lenses are an infection risk so getting them out of the eye as long as possible before surgery reduces this risk.

During The Procedure

LASIK and PRK are quite similar from the patient's perspective though subtle differences between the two exist. Also, the way the flap is made, either with a microkeratome or the femtosecond laser, is slightly different as well. But preparation immediately before the procedure is most likely the same in most refractive surgery facilities. Generally, you will complete the final paperwork upon arrival. Then, you may be offered a low dose of an anti-anxiety medication like Valium. If your doctor has cleared you to take this medication, it can be very helpful. No matter how calm you think you are, most likely adrenaline will be pumping through your system at this point. Within a few minutes after ingestion, Valium can counteract some of the anxiety that all patients experience before any procedure and make it proceed more smoothly. Also, it may make you sleepy after the surgery which is beneficial as we will see.

When the time arrives for your procedure, you will be brought into the laser room. You will then lay on your back on a surgical bed. Your eyes will be prepared for the procedure with a combination of numbing eye drops and probably antibiotic or antiseptic eye drops. Then your eyelids will be cleaned with antiseptic as well. The surgeon will probably cover your eyelids with a drape, a piece of sterile plastic, to keep them out of the way. Once that is done, you are ready for the procedure.

Next, the surgeon will place an instrument called a speculum between the upper and lower eyelids to keep them open. Many patients are concerned they will blink during the surgery, but this cannot happen when the instrument is in place. Also, all patients worry that they will feel pain from the procedure. Since their eyes are numb from drops, however, they will not feel any sensations on the eye during the surgery. However, the eyelids are not numb and can feel the instrument holding the eyelids open. Patients who can relax the muscles around the eye really feel no discomfort at all from the instrument. Other patients involuntarily squeeze their eyes shut as a reflex when things get close to the eyes, so these patients may feel pressure from the instrument holding their eyes open against the squeezing. If they can relax the muscles around the eye, the pressure goes away.

LASIK

When the femtosecond laser is used to create the flap, a suction ring is placed on the eye. This helps keep the eye from moving during flap creation. The suction ring does not cause pain, but some patients describe a mild uncomfortable sensation from it, especially those who reflexively try to squeeze their eyelids shut when the suction is applied. However, the suction is only on the eye for a very short time, usually less than a minute. The femtosecond laser is then docked with the suction ring. The surgeon starts the laser once it is properly centered. The laser is completely painless and only lasts for a few seconds. Most importantly, patients should not move or talk once the laser treatment begins because they can break suction and everything will have to be done all over again.

After the flap is created, the bed is rotated so that the patient is underneath the excimer laser. This is the laser that actually performs the refractive correction. The surgeon will lift the flap and then center the laser on the pupil. Once the laser is locked, it will only treat the area it is supposed to, even if the eye moves slightly. If the eye moves a lot, the treatment will automatically be paused until the eye is brought back into the center. Many patients are concerned that they will move during the treatment, but pupil tracking ensures that the laser treats the appropriate spots even if the eye moves. During treatment, the patient will hear rapid clicking noise and an air aspiration sound like a vacuum cleaner. They may smell a funny odor from the gases emitted by the equipment during the treatment. After treatment is completed, the surgeon will replace the flap and make sure it is aligned properly. This may take a minute or two, and then the treatment is completed for that eye. The whole procedure from start to finish lasts typically less than ten minutes per eye.

The procedure for LASIK with a keratome is very similar to LASIK using the femtosecond laser. A suction ring is also placed on the eye. After proper suction is attained, the keratome is placed on the suction ring and it moves across the eye creating the flap. Again, the suction may be uncomfortable, but patients don't feel the keratome itself because the eye is numb. Once the flap is created, the flap is lifted and the correction performed the same way as described in the paragraph above.

PRK

For PRK, a flap is not created, and so no suction ring is used. Recall that the surface layer of the cornea is the epithelium, which needs to be removed before the excimer laser can do its work. Many different techniques are used to remove it, and all work equally well. Some surgeons use a rotating brush to clean off the epithelium. Others place alcohol on the epithelium to loosen it and then gently brush it away. Removing the epithelium is painless because the eye is numb. When patients involuntarily squeeze their eyes shut, this cause the eye to move a lot, and epithelial removal can take a little longer.

After the epithelium is removed, the excimer laser treatment is performed in the exact same way as described for LASIK in the preceding paragraphs. After the treatment, the surgeon may place an anti-scarring medication on the eye and then will place a bandage contact lens on the eye. The procedure is then complete for that eye.

Post Op

Immediately after the procedure, most surgeons will quickly check each eye before discharging the patient. Plastic shields and/or sunglasses may be used for protection.

After about an hour, the topical anesthetic eye drops will start to wear off, and patients may start to feel discomfort. They may experience excessive tearing, the feeling that something is in their eye, and light sensitivity. Some patients, especially the ones who took Valium right before the procedure, can get home and take a nap before the anesthetic wears off, so they may not experience too much discomfort. Also, if patients can tolerate over-the-counter pain medications like Advil, Motrin, or Aleve, they should take a standard dose right after the procedure to help lessen the discomfort once the anesthetic wears off.

For LASIK patients, once the edges of the flap heal, the pain will diminish quite rapidly. This usually takes only about three to four hours after the procedure. Vision, which may have been somewhat hazy, like being in a steam room, may start to clear up at this time as well. For PRK patients, the whole epithelium has to heal for the pain to go away completely and for vision to clear up. This usually takes twenty-four to forty-eight hours . The most intense discomfort generally lasts for just the first eight hours or so and then becomes pretty tolerable after that until the epithelium heals. For those patients who have breakthrough pain even with the over -the-counter pain medication, the surgeon may prescribe stronger pain medication which is only needed for the first day or two. After your doctor has determined that the epithelium is healed, the bandage contact lenses can be removed.

Once the discomfort is gone, patients will be concerned about their vision. LASIK patients generally have a rapid return to useful vision so that they can drive, read, watch television and perform most daily activities. But it can fluctuate slightly over the first few weeks, maybe night driving will have some glare one night or words on the television may be slightly blurry compared to the day before. PRK patients will take a few extra days to get to useful vision but they too can expect it to fluctuate. Patients should not be concerned about these fluctuations, which are normal and which will lessen over the weeks following the procedure. If the patient is still experiencing some consistently blurry vision, the surgeon may suggest an enhancement to correct any under- or overcorrection that may be present.

Chapter 5: Options in Refractive Surgery

In the early days of laser refractive surgery, patients did not have many choices about how the surgery could be performed. PRK was the only procedure available in the United States. Soon after, flap-making technology improved to the point that LASIK became more popular. As with all things technological, further advances have given us additional options. The more informed you are about *all* the refractive surgery options, the better prepared you will be to make the right choice.

Standard vs. Customized Treatments

The laser that performs the correction for refractive errors needs to be programmed for each patient's prescription. The prescription is based on the eye exam and specifically the refraction. The refraction is that familiar procedure when the doctor or technician has the patient look at an eye chart through a lens device and asks questions like "which is better, one or two?" The patient's answers determine the eyeglass prescription. Certainly, refraction is a skill, and one involving human responses, so its accuracy is prone to human error. Every refraction can be different depending on any number of factors like who performs it or how the patient is feeling that day. Whatever the conditions, when the refraction is used to program the laser, it is usually close enough to get great results in refractive surgery.

However, as one might imagine, some limitations exist with this technique. The obvious one is accuracy. Since the treatment is based on subjective responses, the human factor may cause the correction to be less precise. A less obvious factor has to do with how the treatment pattern is designed.

In a standard treatment, everyone with the same prescription gets the same correction. This is true with glasses and contact lenses as well. Most patients do well with these off-the-shelf corrections. But not every eye is the same. For example, corneal curvatures or overall eye length can vary among patients even if they have the same eyeglass prescription. Some patients experience a degradation of optical quality because of these differences. But what if we could design a treatment that takes them into account?

This is where customized treatments come in. The way customized treatments are designed is extremely complex both optically and mathematically, and an entire book could be written on that subject alone. Anyone, however can understand the basic idea. Remember, in the first chapter on optics when I mentioned that light can be described in different ways, like rays, particles, or waves. Let's think of light as a wave (Figure 23).

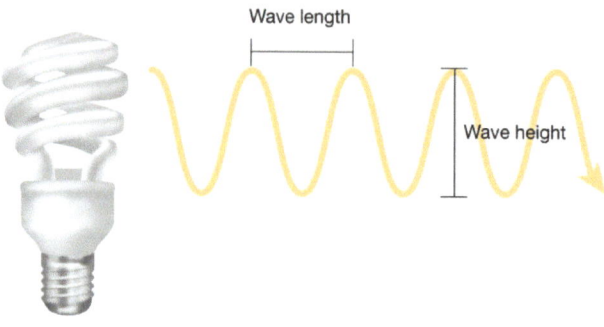

Figure 23: Light exhibits characteristics of waves like length and amplitude or height.

If an optical system has no aberrations, when light is projected into it, the light that reflects out has the same wave shape (Figure 24).

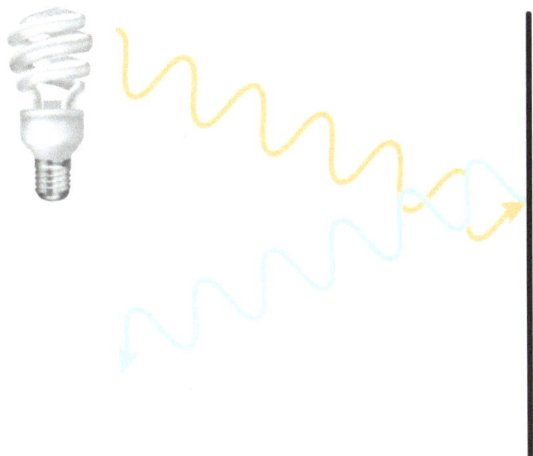

Figure 24: Light reflecting with no aberrations has the same shape.

In an eye with refractive errors, aberrations cause the light waves that reflect out to have a different shape (Figure 25).

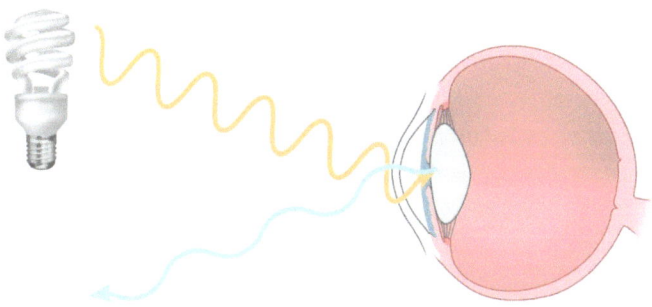

Figure 25: When light reflects out of an eye with refractive errors, the shape of the light waves is different.

The difference in shape between incoming and outgoing light waves is the refractive error of the eye. Customized treatments are designed by an instrument called a wavefront analyzer that shines light of a known wave shape into the eye and then captures the light that is reflected out and measures the new wave shape. The difference between the waves is the refractive error specific for that eye (Figure 26). After measurement, we use a computer to design an ideal treatment that matches the correction.

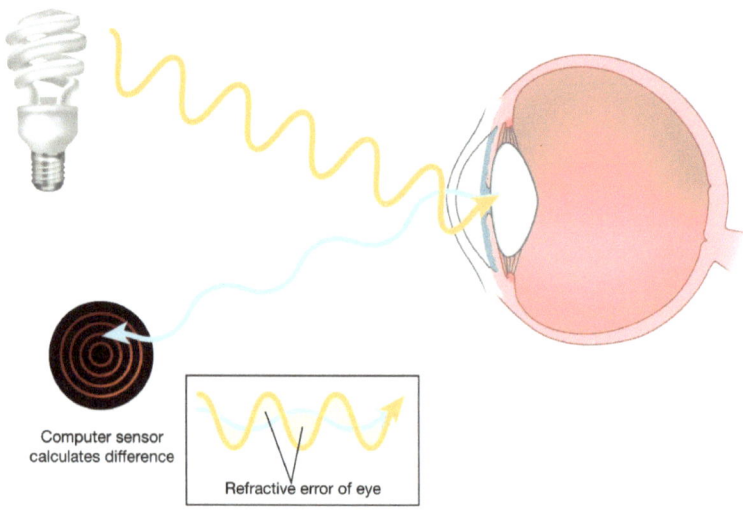

Computer sensor calculates difference

Refractive error of eye

Figure 26: A computer calculates the difference (shaded area) between the incoming lights rays and reflected light rays to calculate the refractive error and to design a customized treatment to correct it.

If you accurately calculate a standard correction, the standard treatment matches most of the correcting wave shape. There will still be, however, a small percentage of the wave better corrected with a customized treatment. Most analyzers show you what extra percent of aberrations, called higher order aberrations, the customization corrects. This can translate into a more accurate correction and also probably decreased night vision disturbances that such aberrations are thought to cause.

So, the question you should ask is, does any of this technology really make a difference? Customized treatments are more costly, so is it worth extra money? Clinically, both standard and custom treatments have extremely high satisfaction rates. Not all patients can have custom treatments because the range of custom treatments available is smaller. For smaller corrections, the difference may be insignificant. In higher corrections though, or in patients with a large astigmatism, custom treatments can lead to better night vision and less chance of needing an enhancement surgery. Custom treatments have automated astigmatism alignment while standard treatments need to be manually aligned. Since each patient is different, you should ask how much the surgeon feels customization will potentially improve your outcome.

Blade vs. Laser Flap

For patients who have LASIK, a flap must be made in the cornea. The first instrument used for flap creation is called a *microkeratome*. It is designed much like a carpenter's plane, and several different models are used today. All of them have gone through years of refinement and improvements, and most surgeons pick one based on preference. Microkeratomes have been used for millions of LASIK procedures and have an excellent track record.

A newer technology using a laser instead of a blade for flap creation was introduced approximately ten years ago. Laser use was slow to catch on at first, mostly because the cost of using it was significantly higher than using a microkeratome. Many surgeons, myself included, were hesitant to pass this cost on to their patients if it did not improve outcomes. When patients hear about "bladeless LASIK," they may think that no cutting is occurring. But a flap has to be made for LASIK, either with a microkeratome or a laser. Much debate has occurred regarding the superiority of one technique over the other. Despite what you might have read or been told, the simple fact is that neither technology is a clear winner. Today, a little over half of all LASIK cases are performed with the laser, and many well-respected surgeons still feel the laser technology just is not worth the extra expense.

I perform LASIK sometimes with a microkeratome and sometimes using the laser for flap creation. I started using the laser because some of my patients asked about it, and I felt I should offer all possible options. Although both procedures have excellent results, I do feel the laser has a slight edge over the microkeratome in several ways. The first is that the flap thickness is much more predictable. This can be important when a patient has a thinner cornea, and the surgeon is trying to preserve as much tissue as possible. The second is that the flap edges are different. With the microkeratome, the flap is tapered in thickness. With the laser, the flap edge is perpendicular to the corneal surface, so the flap fits back into place much like a jigsaw puzzle piece (Figure 27).

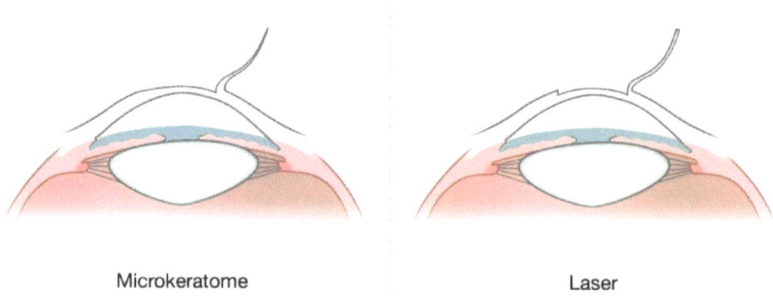

Microkeratome   Laser

Figure 27: The flap edge made with the microkeratome is tapered while the edge from the flap made with the laser is perpendicular.

Therefore, replacing the flap is a little easier with the laser. Finally, flap creation is more controlled with the laser compared to the microkeratome. If an interruption occurs during flap creation, with the laser the surgeon can usually just restart where the interruption occurred. But with the microkeratome, the surgeon usually has to abandon the flap creation.

In some instances, the microkeratome is clearly superior to the laser. The most common advantage is in patients with corneal scars. If the patient has a scar, say from a prior infection, the laser does not penetrate well, sometimes resulting in an irregular flap. Scars usually do not present a problem for the microkeratome. Also, some feel the corneal bed under the flap is smoother with a microkeratome compared to the laser. Since my personal preference is to use the laser, I usually advise patients to use it if they can. But if the extra expense is an issue, I reassure them that using the microkeratome is still a great alternative and by no means an obsolete technique. Since each case is different, you should discuss with your surgeon how each one can benefit you.

Conclusion

I hope you have found this introduction to refractive surgery useful. If you have not yet had an evaluation by your local refractive surgeon, this information may help in understanding the information presented during the consultation. At the very least, it should have provoked lots of good questions for your doctor. It may also help make sense of the concepts after the consult as well. If you have additional questions, I encourage you to contact me via our website, www.palisadeslaser.com, or email me at rgordon@ramapoeyecare.com.

About The Author

Richard N. Gordon, M.D., is the founder and Medical Director of the Palisades Laser Eye Center located in Pomona, NY. He graduated *cum laude* from Amherst College and attended medical school at New York University. He interned at St. Raphael's/Yale University and completed his ophthalmology residency at Montefiore Medical Center. He completed his fellowship at the New York Eye and Ear Infirmary in Manhattan and is currently Associate Adjunct Professor of Ophthalmology there. He has performed thousands of refractive procedures since the laser center's opening in 1999.

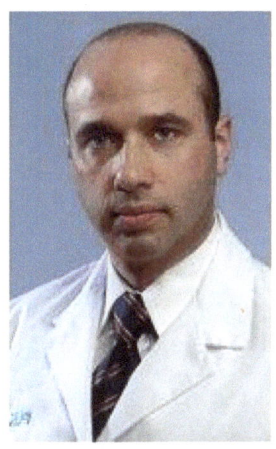

www.ingramcontent.com/pod-product-compliance
Lightning Source LLC
Chambersburg PA
CBHW040855180526
45159CB00001B/429